I0830425

Conversations with a Nutritionist

Health
Nutrition
& Lifestyle

Your way back to Good Health!

I am a 45 year old person, 175 cm tall, 82 kg weight, of average physical fitness and no medical conditions. You being an expert nutritionist and fitness expert, kindly give me guidance on the following enquiries related with health, fitness and nutrition.

1. What would be "prime of health" for me and what all do I need to do for the same?

The 'prime of health' for someone in your age and physical condition would include a balanced diet that is rich in whole grains, lean proteins, fruits, and vegetables. It is also important to stay active and get enough exercise to maintain a healthy weight. Regular physical activity, such as brisk walking, jogging, swimming, or biking, will help to keep your heart and lungs in good shape. Additionally, it is important to get enough sleep and reduce stress levels. Lastly, it is a good idea to get regular check-ups with your doctor to ensure that any underlying medical conditions are caught early.

2. What kind of diet should I follow?

A diet that is rich in whole grains, lean proteins, fruits, and vegetables is ideal. It is important to avoid processed and sugary foods, as well as foods that are high in saturated fats. Eating a variety of foods will help ensure that you get all the vitamins and minerals your body needs. Additionally, it is important to drink plenty of water throughout the day to stay properly hydrated.

3. What kind of exercise should I do to maintain my physical fitness?

Regular physical activity is important for maintaining physical fitness. Brisk walking, jogging, swimming, and biking are all great forms of exercise that will help to keep your heart and lungs in good shape. Additionally, strength training exercises, such as lifting weights, can help to build muscle and improve your overall fitness level. It is important to choose activities that you enjoy, as this will make it easier to stick to your exercise routine.

4. What lifestyle changes should I make to live a healthier life?

Making lifestyle changes to live a healthier life is an important part of overall health. Eating a balanced diet and getting regular exercise are both essential for maintaining good health. Additionally, it is important to get enough sleep, reduce stress levels, and to avoid smoking and excessive alcohol consumption. Making small changes to your lifestyle, such as eating more fruits and vegetables, can make a big difference in your overall health and well-being.

Give me a meal plan for maintaining ideal bodyweight and getting all nutrients naturally

Breakfast: Oatmeal with banana, blueberries, and walnuts.

Snack: Yogurt with berries, nuts, and a sprinkle of granola.

Lunch: Salad with grilled chicken, feta cheese, and a light vinaigrette.

Snack: Hummus with carrots and celery.

Dinner: Salmon over quinoa with steamed vegetables.

Snack: Fruit smoothie with almond milk, banana, and spinach.

Give me a meal plan of common Indian cuisine with ingredients that are commonly used in Indian cooking.

Breakfast: Poha (flattened rice) with vegetables, peanuts, and lime.

Snack: Aloo Tikki (potato patties) with chutney.

Lunch: Dal (lentil stew) with rice, roti (flatbread), and a vegetable side dish.

Snack: Pani puri (filled pastry shells) with tamarind chutney.

Dinner: Vegetable biryani (rice dish) with raita (yogurt dip).

Snack: Jalebi (deep-fried pastry) with milk.

What would be the calorie count of the above given Indian cuisine meal plan.

The calorie count for the given Indian cuisine meal plan would depend on the exact ingredients and amounts used for each dish. Generally speaking, the breakfast and snack options would be approximately 400-500 calories each, the lunch and dinner options would be around 500-700 calories each, and the snack options would be around 200-300 calories each. Modify this meal plan to have a total of approx 1500 calories in a day. The plan should include 90 gms protein and required fiber intake for a 45 year old Indian male.

Breakfast: Oatmeal with banana, almond milk, and walnuts (300 calories, 10g protein, 5g fiber)
Snack: Yogurt with berries, nuts, and a sprinkle of granola (400 calories, 10g protein, 3g fiber)

Lunch: Dal (lentil stew) with rice, roti (flatbread), and a vegetable side dish (600 calories, 25g protein, 10g fiber)
Snack: Hummus with carrots and celery (200 calories, 6g protein, 4g fiber)

Dinner: Grilled chicken over quinoa with steamed vegetables (500 calories, 25g protein, 5g fiber)
Snack: Fruit smoothie with almond milk, banana, and spinach (200 calories, 5g protein, 3g fiber)

Please mention measurable amount of all the ingredients of the above suggested diet plan.

Breakfast:
- 1/2 cup oatmeal
- 1/2 banana
- 1/2 cup almond milk
- 1 tablespoon walnuts

Snack:
- 1/2 cup yogurt
- 1/4 cup berries
- 1 tablespoon nuts
- 1 tablespoon granola

Lunch:
- 1/2 cup dal
- 1/2 cup rice
- 1 roti
- 1/2 cup vegetable side dish

Snack:
- 1/4 cup hummus
- 1/2 cup carrots
- 1/2 cup celery

Dinner:
- 1/2 cup grilled chicken
- 1/2 cup quinoa
- 1 cup steamed vegetables

Snack:
- 1 cup fruit smoothie
- 1/2 cup almond milk
- 1/2 banana
- 1/2 cup spinach

Define the cup volume in ml ?

- A cup is equal to 8 fluid ounces, or 236.6 milliliters.

Please suggest Indian substitute (with quantity) for the following:
- **1/2 cup almond milk**
- **1/2 cup yogurt**
- **1/4 cup berries**
- **1 tablespoon nuts**
- **1 tablespoon granola**
- **1/4 cup hummus**
- **1/2 cup carrots**
- **1/2 cup celery**
- **1/2 cup quinoa**
- **1 cup steamed vegetables**
- **1 cup fruit smoothie**
- **1/2 cup almond milk**
- **1/2 cup spinach**

- 1/2 cup almond milk - Substitute: 1/2 cup coconut milk
- 1/2 cup yogurt - Substitute: 1/2 cup lassi
- 1/4 cup berries - Substitute: 1/4 cup chopped mango
- 1 tablespoon nuts - Substitute: 1 tablespoon roasted chana dal
- 1 tablespoon granola - Substitute: 1 tablespoon muesli
- 1/4 cup hummus - Substitute: 1/4 cup chutney
- 1/2 cup carrots - Substitute: 1/2 cup grated bottle gourd
- 1/2 cup celery - Substitute: 1/2 cup chopped spinach
- 1/2 cup quinoa - Substitute: 1/2 cup cooked basmati rice
- 1 cup steamed vegetables - Substitute: 1 cup cooked mixed vegetables

- 1 cup fruit smoothie - Substitute: 1 cup lassi
- 1/2 cup almond milk - Substitute: 1/2 cup coconut milk
- 1/2 cup spinach - Substitute: 1/2 cup cooked palak paneer

Please suggest further some more indian substitute (with quantity) for the following

- 1/2 cup almond milk - Substitute: 1/2 cup coconut milk
- 1/4 cup berries - Substitute: 1/4 cup chopped mango
- 1 tablespoon granola - Substitute: 1 tablespoon muesli
- 1/4 cup hummus - Substitute: 1/4 cup chutney
- 1/2 cup celery - Substitute: 1/2 cup chopped spinach
- 1/2 cup quinoa - Substitute: 1/2 cup cooked basmati rice
- 1 cup fruit smoothie - Substitute: 1 cup lassi
- 1/2 cup almond milk - Substitute: 1/2 cup coconut milk

- 1/2 cup almond milk - Substitute: 1/2 cup almond-coconut milk
- 1/4 cup berries - Substitute: 1/4 cup chopped pineapple
- 1 tablespoon granola - Substitute: 1 tablespoon oats
- 1/4 cup hummus - Substitute: 1/4 cup peanut butter
- 1/2 cup celery - Substitute: 1/2 cup chopped tomato
- 1/2 cup quinoa - Substitute: 1/2 cup cooked brown rice
- 1 cup fruit smoothie - Substitute: 1 cup mango lassi
- 1/2 cup almond milk - Substitute: 1/2 cup almond-coconut milk

Please suggest ways to increase cardio respiratory fitness, muscle strength, aerobic endurance, flexibility, balance, agility, reaction time, and power in a 45 year old Indian Male, 175 cm tall, 82 kg weight, of average physical fitness and no medical conditions.

Cardio respiratory Fitness:
- Brisk walking, jogging, swimming, or biking
- High-intensity interval training

Muscle Strength:
- Weight lifting
- Resistance bands
- Bodyweight exercises

Aerobic Endurance:
- Running
- Cycling
- Swimming

Flexibility:
- Stretching
- Yoga
- Pilates

Balance:
- Single-leg exercises
- Standing on a balance board
- Yoga poses

Agility:
• Ladder drills
• Jumping rope
• Side shuffling

Reaction Time:
• Reaction drills
• Plyometric drills
• Agility drills

Power:
• Plyometric exercises
• Medicine ball throws
• Sprints
• Jump squats

How much time would I need to be in good physical shape on the above parameters if I give it 45 minutes daily for 5 days every week.

It is difficult to say how long it would take to reach a good level of physical fitness, as this will depend on individual factors such as age, current fitness level, and health. Generally speaking, it could take anywhere from 6 to 12 weeks of consistent effort to see noticeable changes in physical fitness. However, with a commitment to 45 minutes of exercise 5 days a week and a healthy diet, you should see improvements in your overall fitness level within a few weeks.

I can commit to a daily 45-60 minutes of exercise 5 days a week.

Incorporating the above suggestions, can you please give me a 12 weeks (03 months) fitness activity plan with the schedule week wise mentioning each activity with duration.

Week 1:
Monday: 30 minutes of brisk walking + 15 minutes of stretching
Tuesday: 30 minutes of biking + 15 minutes of strength training
Wednesday: 30 minutes of swimming + 15 minutes of agility drills
Thursday: 30 minutes of jogging + 15 minutes of balance exercises
Friday: 30 minutes of running + 15 minutes of plyometric exercises
Saturday: 30 minutes of weight lifting + 15 minutes of reaction drills
Sunday: Rest

Week 2:
Monday: 30 minutes of brisk walking + 15 minutes of stretching
Tuesday: 30 minutes of biking + 15 minutes of strength training
Wednesday: 30 minutes of swimming + 15 minutes of agility drills
Thursday: 30 minutes of jogging + 15 minutes of balance exercises

Friday: 30 minutes of running + 15 minutes of plyometric exercises

Saturday: 30 minutes of weight lifting + 15 minutes of reaction drills

Sunday: 30 minutes of yoga + 15 minutes of jump rope

Week 3:

Monday: 30 minutes of brisk walking + 15 minutes of stretching

Tuesday: 30 minutes of biking + 15 minutes of strength training

Wednesday: 30 minutes of swimming + 15 minutes of agility drills

Thursday: 30 minutes of jogging + 15 minutes of balance exercises

Friday: 30 minutes of running + 15 minutes of plyometric exercises

Saturday: 30 minutes of weight lifting + 15 minutes of reaction drills

Sunday: 30 minutes of yoga + 15 minutes of jump rope

Week 4:

Monday: 30 minutes of brisk walking + 15 minutes of stretching

Tuesday: 30 minutes of biking + 15 minutes of strength training

Wednesday: 30 minutes of swimming + 15 minutes of agility drills

Thursday: 30 minutes of jogging + 15 minutes of balance exercises

Friday: 30 minutes of running + 15 minutes of plyometric exercises
Saturday: 30 minutes of weight lifting + 15 minutes of reaction drills
Sunday: 30 minutes of yoga + 15 minutes of jump rope

Week 5:
Monday: 30 minutes of brisk walking + 15 minutes of stretching
Tuesday: 30 minutes of biking + 15 minutes of strength training
Wednesday: 30 minutes of swimming + 15 minutes of agility drills
Thursday: 30 minutes of jogging + 15 minutes of balance exercises
Friday: 30 minutes of running + 15 minutes of plyometric exercises
Saturday: 30 minutes of weight lifting + 15 minutes of reaction drills
Sunday: Rest

Week 6:
Monday: 30 minutes of brisk walking + 15 minutes of stretching
Tuesday: 30 minutes of biking + 15 minutes of strength training
Wednesday: 30 minutes of swimming + 15 minutes of agility drills
Thursday: 30 minutes of jogging + 15 minutes of balance exercises

Friday: 30 minutes of running + 15 minutes of plyometric exercises
Saturday: 30 minutes of weight lifting + 15 minutes of reaction drills
Sunday: 30 minutes of yoga + 15 minutes of jump rope

Week 7:
Monday: 30 minutes of brisk walking + 15 minutes of stretching
Tuesday: 30 minutes of biking + 15 minutes of strength training
Wednesday: 30 minutes of swimming + 15 minutes of agility drills
Thursday: 30 minutes of jogging + 15 minutes of balance exercises
Friday: 30 minutes of running + 15 minutes of plyometric exercises
Saturday: 30 minutes of weight lifting + 15 minutes of reaction drills
Sunday: 30 minutes of yoga + 15 minutes of jump rope

Week 8:
Monday: 30 minutes of brisk walking + 15 minutes of stretching
Tuesday: 30 minutes of biking + 15 minutes of strength training
Wednesday: 30 minutes of swimming + 15 minutes of agility drills
Thursday: 30 minutes of jogging + 15 minutes of balance exercises

Friday: 30 minutes of running + 15 minutes of plyometric exercises
Saturday: 30 minutes of weight lifting + 15 minutes of reaction drills
Sunday: Rest

Week 9:
Monday: 30 minutes of brisk walking + 15 minutes of stretching
Tuesday: 30 minutes of biking + 15 minutes of strength training
Wednesday: 30 minutes of swimming + 15 minutes of agility drills
Thursday: 30 minutes of jogging + 15 minutes of balance exercises
Friday: 30 minutes of running + 15 minutes of plyometric exercises
Saturday: 30 minutes of weight lifting + 15 minutes of reaction drills
Sunday: 30 minutes of yoga + 15 minutes of jump rope

Week 10:
Monday: 30 minutes of brisk walking + 15 minutes of stretching
Tuesday: 30 minutes of biking + 15 minutes of strength training
Wednesday: 30 minutes of swimming + 15 minutes of agility drills
Thursday: 30 minutes of jogging + 15 minutes of balance exercises

Friday: 30 minutes of running + 15 minutes of plyometric exercises
Saturday: 30 minutes of weight lifting + 15 minutes of reaction drills
Sunday: 30 minutes of yoga + 15 minutes of jump rope

Week 11:
Monday: 30 minutes of brisk walking + 15 minutes of stretching
Tuesday: 30 minutes of biking + 15 minutes of strength training
Wednesday: 30 minutes of swimming + 15 minutes of agility drills
Thursday: 30 minutes of jogging + 15 minutes of balance exercises
Friday: 30 minutes of running + 15 minutes of plyometric exercises
Saturday: 30 minutes of weight lifting + 15 minutes of reaction drills
Sunday: Rest

Week 12:
Monday: 30 minutes of brisk walking + 15 minutes of stretching
Tuesday: 30 minutes of biking + 15 minutes of strength training
Wednesday: 30 minutes of swimming + 15 minutes of agility drills
Thursday: 30 minutes of jogging + 15 minutes of balance exercises

Friday: 30 minutes of running + 15 minutes of plyometric exercises

Saturday: 30 minutes of weight lifting + 15 minutes of reaction drills

Sunday: 30 minutes of yoga + 15 minutes of jump rope

Can you give details of the following covering each one in details

15 minutes of agility drills
15 minutes of balance exercises
15 minutes of plyometric exercises
15 minutes of reaction drills

Agility Drills:
• Ladder drills: Running through a ladder laid on the ground with quick side shuffles and high knees
• Hops: Jumping forward and backward over an obstacle or line
• Zig-Zags: Running in a zig-zag motion through a set of cones

Balance Exercises:
• Single-Leg Balance: Standing on one foot and holding the other in the air for 30 seconds
• Balance Board: Standing on a balance board with feet shoulder-width apart and arms outstretched
• Yoga Poses: Tree pose, warrior pose, and mountain pose

Plyometric Exercises:
• Squat Jumps: Jumping with legs bent and feet together, then landing softly with knees bent
• Jump Squats: Squatting down and then jumping as high as possible
• Medicine Ball Throws: Throwing a medicine ball up against a wall and catching it

Reaction Drills:

• Reaction Ball: Throwing a reaction ball against a wall and catching it
• Plyometric Drills: Jumping up and down and side to side over an obstacle or line
• Agility

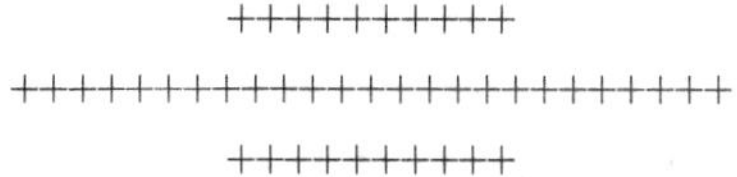

Give me guidance on What lifestyle changes should I make to live a healthier life?

1. Eat a balanced diet:
2. Exercise regularly:
3. Get adequate sleep:
4. Reduce stress:
5. Drink plenty of water:
6. Manage alcohol intake:
7. Avoid smoking:
8. Take time for yourself:

Please elaborate…

1. Eat a Balanced Diet:

Eating a balanced diet is essential for maintaining overall health and wellbeing. A balanced diet consists of foods from all the food groups, including fruits, vegetables, whole grains, lean proteins, and healthy fats. Fruits and vegetables are rich in antioxidants, vitamins, and minerals. Whole grains provide dietary fiber and are a good source of energy. Lean proteins such as fish, poultry, and beans provide essential amino acids and help build and repair muscles. Healthy fats, such as those found in nuts, seeds, and avocados, provide essential fatty acids and help to regulate hormones. Processed and refined foods should be limited as they are low in nutrients and high in calories and additives.

Eating a balanced diet helps to ensure that you are getting all the vitamins, minerals, and nutrients you need to maintain optimal health. It also helps to regulate your blood sugar, reduce inflammation, and protect against chronic diseases such as heart disease, diabetes, and cancer. Additionally, eating a balanced diet can help to improve mental clarity and reduce stress.

When planning your meals, aim for variety and moderation. Eat a variety of foods from each food group and aim for about 25-35% of your total calorie intake to come from healthy fats, 20-35% from proteins, and 45-65% from carbohydrates. Additionally, it is important to pay attention to portion sizes and opt for smaller portions when possible. Eating smaller, more frequent meals can be beneficial for maintaining energy levels and avoiding overeating.

Finally, it is important to pay attention to your body's hunger signals. Eat when you are hungry and stop when you are full. Don't feel obligated to finish every meal, or to eat when you are not hungry. Eating should be an enjoyable experience, not a chore.

2. Exercise Regularly:

Exercise is an important part of a healthy lifestyle. Regular physical activity helps to promote physical and mental health and can have numerous benefits, including weight management, improved cardiovascular health, and improved mood. Aim for at least 30 minutes of physical activity at least 5 days a week. Choose activities that you enjoy, such as walking, jogging, swimming, cycling, or any other form of exercise.

Cardiovascular exercise, such as running, biking, and swimming, is great for boosting heart health and improving endurance. Strength training, such as using weights or bodyweight exercises, can help to build and maintain muscle mass, improve posture, and reduce age-related muscle loss. Flexibility exercises, such as stretching, yoga, or pilates, can help to improve range of motion and reduce the risk of injury.

In addition to regular exercise, it is important to make time for rest and recovery. Incorporate at least one day of rest into your schedule each week and take breaks between exercise sessions. Make sure to stretch before and after exercise to reduce the risk of injury. Additionally, make sure to wear appropriate clothing and footwear and stay properly hydrated throughout your workouts.

Exercising regularly can have numerous benefits, including improving overall physical health, boosting energy levels, and improving mental clarity. Exercise can also help to reduce stress, improve sleep, and enhance overall wellbeing. So make sure to make time for physical activity each day and enjoy the many benefits of regular exercise.

3. Get Adequate Sleep:

Getting adequate sleep is essential for maintaining overall health and wellbeing. Sleep is necessary for physical and mental recovery, and it helps to regulate hormones, boost immunity, and improve cognitive function. Aim for 7-8 hours of sleep per night to ensure that your body is well-rested and your mind is alert.

There are a few things you can do to improve your sleep quality. Try to stick to a regular sleep schedule and go to bed and wake up at the same time each day. Avoid caffeine and other stimulants late in the day, as they can interfere with sleep. Exercise regularly, but not too close to bedtime. Additionally, create a relaxing bedtime routine that helps to prepare your body for sleep. This could include taking a warm bath, reading a book, or practicing relaxation techniques.

If you are having difficulty falling asleep, try avoiding screens at least an hour before bed. The blue light emitted by screens can disrupt your body's natural sleep-wake cycle. Additionally, try to avoid napping during the day, as this can make it difficult to fall asleep at night.

Getting enough sleep is essential for maintaining overall health and wellbeing. It helps to regulate hormones, boost immunity, and improve cognitive function. So make sure to get 7-8 hours of quality sleep each night to ensure that your body and mind are well-rested and alert.

4. Reduce Stress:

Reducing stress is essential for maintaining overall health and wellbeing. Stress can take a toll on both physical and mental health, and can lead to a number of issues, such as insomnia, digestive problems, depression, and anxiety. Take time to relax and engage in activities that help to reduce stress.

Practicing mindfulness can be helpful for reducing stress. Mindfulness is a form of meditation that focuses on being present in the moment and observing your thoughts and feelings without judgment. Additionally, spending time in nature can help to reduce stress. Nature walks or hikes can be a great way to relax and clear your mind.

Yoga and tai chi are also great activities for reducing stress. Both involve gentle movements and breathing exercises that can help to relax the body and clear the mind. Additionally, massage therapy is great for reducing stress and tension in the body.

Finally, take time for activities that bring you joy. Whether it's reading a book, listening to music, or engaging in a hobby, make sure to take time for yourself. Doing things you enjoy can help to reduce stress and improve overall wellbeing.

Reducing stress is essential for maintaining physical and mental health. Take time to relax

5. Drink Plenty of Water:

Staying hydrated is essential for overall health and wellbeing. Water helps to flush out toxins, regulate body temperature, and lubricate joints and organs. Additionally, it helps to regulate appetite and boost metabolism. Aim to drink at least 8 glasses of water per day.

When choosing beverages, opt for water whenever possible. Coffee, tea, and other caffeinated beverages should be limited as they can act as diuretics and cause dehydration. Additionally, limit sugary drinks such as sodas, juices, and sports drinks.

If you find it difficult to drink enough water, try to incorporate it into your daily routine. Carry a reusable water bottle with you throughout the day and aim to finish it by the end of the day. Additionally, add flavor to your water by adding slices of citrus fruits, cucumber, or herbs such as mint or basil.

Staying hydrated is essential for overall health and wellbeing. Aim to drink at least 8 glasses of water per day to ensure that your body is well-hydrated and functioning optimally.

6. Manage Alcohol Intake:

If you choose to drink alcohol, do so in moderation. Excessive alcohol consumption can take a toll on your health and wellbeing. The Dietary Guidelines for Americans recommend no more than 2 drinks per day for men and 1 drink per day for women.

Alcohol is a diuretic, meaning it causes your body to lose more fluids than it takes in. Therefore, it is important to stay hydrated when drinking alcohol. Have a glass of water in between each alcoholic drink and try to limit your intake to no more than 2 drinks per day.

Alcohol can also interfere with sleep and impair cognitive function. Therefore, it is best to avoid drinking too close to bedtime and to limit your alcohol intake if you have to be active the next day. Additionally, drinking alcohol can impair judgement and increase the risk of injury. It is especially important to drink responsibly if you are in a new environment or unfamiliar situation.

If you choose to drink alcohol, do so in moderation. Excessive alcohol consumption can take a toll on your health and wellbeing. So be mindful of your alcohol intake and always drink responsibly.

7. Avoid Smoking:

Smoking is detrimental to your health. Smoking can damage your lungs, increase your risk of heart disease, and increase your risk of cancer. If you smoke, quit as soon as possible.

If you are trying to quit smoking, there are a few things you can do to make quitting easier. First, make a plan. Set a quit date and create a list of strategies that will help you reach your goal. Then, identify your triggers and make a plan to avoid or manage them.

Second, reach out for help and support. There are many resources available to help you quit smoking. Your doctor can provide advice on quitting strategies, and there are numerous support groups and online communities to provide encouragement and advice.

Finally, reward yourself. Celebrate your achievements and reward yourself with non-smoking related activities. This could include treating yourself to a massage, going to a movie, or spending time with friends.

Smoking is detrimental to your health, so it is important to quit as soon as possible. Make a plan, reach out for help, and reward yourself for your successes.

8. Take Time for Yourself:

Taking time for yourself is essential for maintaining overall health and wellbeing. Make sure to take time each day to do activities that bring you joy. This could include reading a book, listening to music, or engaging in a hobby.

Taking time for yourself can help to reduce stress, improve mood, and enhance overall wellbeing. Additionally, it can help to improve focus and increase productivity.

When taking time for yourself, it is important to focus on activities that bring you joy. This could include listening to your favorite music, taking a relaxing walk in nature, or engaging in a hobby. Additionally, it is important to make time for social activities. Spend time with friends, family, or loved ones, or join a club or group to meet new people.

Finally, make sure to take time for yourself each day. Whether it's 10 minutes or a few hours, make sure to take time to do activities that bring you joy and improve your overall wellbeing.

++++++++++

End ! 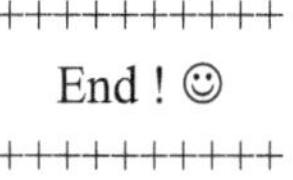

++++++++++